LOVE ME BACK TO HEALTH
"LOVE NEVER FAILS"

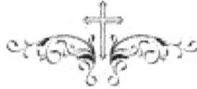

"Amazing Exposition of what the Church Needs Most - Agape LOVE"

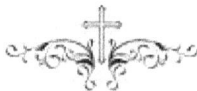

AUTHOR

MARY RIEVES

LOVE ME BACK TO HEALTH

Mary Rieves is available to conduct conferences, seminars, and webinars. This publication is available for educational purposes at special quantity discounts.

CONTACT
Pastor Mary Rieves
www.maryrievesministries.com
maryrievesministries@yahoo.com
Kogichurch@yahoo.com
813-501-3217

Editing
MTN Consulting, Bradenton, Florida/TAGIN, INC Tampa

Cover Design & Book Design
TAGIN, INC Tampa Florida

Photographs
The Olive Tree Photography Company, Tampa, Florida

All Bible Quotes and Scripture References
King James Version (KJV)
Amplified Version
Message Version

Printed in the United States of America

~TABLE OF CONTENTS~

~FOREWORD~

It indeed takes a call to write such a book as "Love Me Back To Health" with a plethora of daily activities to move you away from writing. Even more to write about your own life experiences and share with the world.

This is what Pastor Mary is doing taking us through the many corridors of her life with real life people. Pastor Mary has overcome a lot of obstacles in her life and let others read and know the same God that "Loved her Back to Health" will be the same God to love you even as you read this book. And while we don't fully know everything about ourselves or our future, we do know that within the corridors of our heart are very dark rooms that have been closed to the public until we face them privately. There are places that we fear to enter in and only hear stories about like the one you are about to read.

Pastor Mary drives home her points, not from a "reality show" but from the show of realization that Jesus loves us infinitely. That He gave Himself for you and me. He laid down His life for us to live our best life totally healed. It is the kind of love that sees our vulnerability, knows our brokenness and comes to see about us. This book page by page chapter by chapter will reveal to you the love of our Father which art in heaven. Take, eat ye all of it.

Dr. Brenda Fruster
WINNER'S Worship Center
Tampa, Florida

~

~ACKNOWLEDGEMENTS~

I dedicate this book to my parents, the late Bishop T. J. Rogers and Prophetess Tallie Ann Rogers. Thank you for teaching us how to love and show kindness to others. You both have been such powerful and great examples in our lives. I did not understand how you could love people who mistreated you. Now I understand; it is the love of Jesus Christ that constrained you.

You refused to allow other to shake your focus. Instead, you focused on your destinies and your job to prepare an inheritance for your children.

Thank you for raising us up in the way of the Lord, and for teaching us right from wrong. I remember you admonishing that God was not pleased with what we were doing. You made sure your house was in order before you went to the church. For this, I would like to say thank you.

Mom, thank you for showing me how to be a true woman of God and to not make excuses for my mistakes. You never blamed others for your problems or mistakes. Although you and Dad had rough childhoods, you made sure we had a wonderful life. You taught us, "You do not have to become what others see you as now," and "you will become what God had ordained you to be!"

Dad, I remember your stories about how you were drunk all of the time, until the day one of the mothers asked to pray for you. Even though you were intoxicated as you made your way the front of the church, God immediately transformed your life! I personally never witnessed you drinking and never saw you drunk. Thank God that I witnessed how powerful you were in God as you matriculated from husband to dad, friend to pastor, and doctor to a Bishop. Rest on Dad. We have not forgotten you and we love you much!

Continue to prophesy Mom, even when people do not want to hear it, or cannot comprehend that the Word of God brings life or death. You once reprimanded me for having a bad attitude and I responded that I did not have a bad attitude. I now admit that my attitude was bad, but God had His way of handling that.

I pray that we have made you and Dad proud of us. I am proud of my brothers and sisters and thankful for our gifts received from God. A promise was made concerning your seed, and we are walking in that promise. Continue to pray for us. We all love you very much. Mom, enjoy this book!

To my husband & Pastor, Darrell Rieves: Thank you for supporting me in all that I do. Praise God for allowing you to find me, a little country girl—a cute little country girl! Thank you for being a good husband, father, son, brother, and friend. I know that at times I get on your nerves, but we were made for each other. Everything we have gone through has been for purpose. I am glad that God has allowed us to walk and travel this journey together. You have grown so much from the time I met you, and I pray that you see growth in me. Keep your hands in God's hands and never let go. You were the one who prophesied these books, so to you I say, "thank you." This is number two!

To my beloved children, Joshua, Naomi, and Rachel and my Glam Babies, Thank you, for putting up with your mother. I am proud of you all. Never forget that you can do all things through Christ that strengthens you! I love you all very much.

To my brothers and sisters: Thank you for your strong support. This family is like no other family, and I am so happy to be a part of it. I thank God that we recognize and respect the gifts of God in each other. Continue to do the will of God and never let go of His hands. Let's continue supporting each other, and teach our children—just as our parents have taught us. A special thanks to my sister Barbara Mitchell for believing in me! We may laugh about what we do and the vision God gives us, but we totally believe in each other! You've helped to push me into my destiny.' Thank you for hanging in there with me. We have worked together for such a long time, and it has been wonderful getting under your wings and watching as God uses us! Powerful!

To Kingdom of God International Church: I love you all and am eternally grateful for your support! Our ministry was founded on LOVE! Words cannot express how happy I am that God entrusted Pastor Darrell and I to lead such great people. Ms. Bea, thank you for your continue support to assist me! I love you all! KOGIC is the place to be!

To Bishop and First Lady Warren: Thank you for being powerful examples, and for taking Darrell and I to the next level of our destinies! You took us in as if we were your own and for this we say, "Thank you!"

To Bishop and First Lady James E. Holloway, Sr.: Thank you for seeing beyond my NOW! Because of you, I am walking in places I could only dream of. I love you Bishop and Lady Holloway!

To my editor, Detra Moore Brown: You are an angel sent from heaven! Words cannot express how much I thank God for you and your ability to do what you do.

Annie Avery, my sister from another mother! I am forever grateful to you! You always have had my back. I LOVE YOU!

Pastor Sherry Major, Pastor Brenda Fruster and Bishop Marcus McIntosh, I bless God for each of you! You have no idea the impact you have made in my life. I am so honored to know you all. What great examples you are to the body of Christ. Thank you!

To all my family and friends: Thank you so much for always supporting Mary Rieves Ministries.

To my girl Marinda Carter, oh how I miss you! I dedicate this book to you my girl!!!

~

I.   1 Corinthians 13:4-10(MSG)

[3-7] If I give everything I own to the poor and even go to the stake to be burned as a martyr, but I don't love, I've gotten nowhere. So, no matter what I say, what I believe, and what I do, I'm bankrupt without love.

Love never gives up.
Love cares more for others than for self.
Love doesn't want what it doesn't have.
Love doesn't strut,
Doesn't have a swelled head,
Doesn't force itself on others,
Isn't always "me first,"
Doesn't fly off the handle,
Doesn't keep score of the sins of others,
Doesn't revel when others grovel,
Takes pleasure in the flowering of truth,
Puts up with anything,
Trusts God always,
Always looks for the best,
Never looks back,
But keeps going to the end.

[8-10] *Love never dies. Inspired speech will be over some day; praying in tongues will end; understanding will reach its limit. We know only a portion of the truth, and what we say about God is always incomplete. But when the Complete arrives, our incompletes will be canceled.*

WHY I WROTE THIS BOOK

God told me that the most important thing the church is missing is LOVE! I am not referring to the different types of love we hear about and "experience" throughout our lives. I am talking about a deep and abiding love that only God can give. A type of love that will change a life forever. After you operate in this Love, all other types are superficial and meaningless. This love is the one and only LOVE we all should possess and operate in. It is Agape LOVE! This is the Love of Christ, unconditional love.

Type of Loves we know:

* Eros or sexual passion. The first kind of love was Eros, named after the Greek god of fertility, and it represented the idea of sexual passion and desire. ...
* Philia or deep friendship. ...
* Ludus or playful love. ...
* *Agape or love for everyone, which is God's love. ...*
* Pragma or longstanding love. ...
* Philautia or love of the self.

There are times that people may make us mad, sometimes we are not in agreement with their lifestyle or they refuse to do what is asked of them; this may cause us to stop "loving" them. This is not the way to handle things according to the word of God. When we change the way we treat people, it causes them to separate or draw closer to us. Even when I don't agree with someone, mistreated by them, even when they lie on me, even when they steal from me and if they try to kill my character; I still have to display the Love of Christ at all time.

We are very quick to judge one another and we forget that we all fall short sometimes.

I love what John 3:16-18 (MSG) says,

16-18 "This is how much God loved the world: He gave his Son, his one and only Son. And this is why: so that no one need be destroyed; by believing in him, anyone can have a whole and lasting life. God didn't go to all the trouble of sending his Son merely to point an accusing finger, telling the world how bad it was. He came to help, to put the world right again. Anyone who trusts in him is acquitted; anyone who refuses to trust him has long since been under the death sentence without knowing it. And why? Because of that person's failure to believe in the one-of-a-kind Son of God when introduced to him.

Take a moment with John 3:16-18. Read it again! What are the key sentences in these scriptures?

    a. He Loved Us So Much
    b. He Gave His Only Son
    c. No One Need To Be Destroyed
    d. You Can Have Everlasting Life
    e. He Did Not Send his Son To Point An Accusing Finger
    f. He Came To Help Put The World Back Right Again
    g. Anyone Who TRUSTS in HIM is ACQUITTED!

h. Anyone Who Refuses To TRUST HIM is under
    the DEATH SENTENCE WITHOUT
    KNOWING IT

The above is very important to remember because it
illustrates God's plan for mankind and agape love. Through
it, we remind ourselves why God sent his only Son into this
world. He created a path for a sinful people to experience
external life through Jesus. This is so powerful because it lets
us know that God loved us so much that he would not give
up on us even when he should have. What a powerful
example of how we should never give up on anyone. The
Father, Son and the Holy Ghost have given us POWER to
Love people back to health!

~CHAPTER 1~

<u>GOD'S LOVE FOR US</u>

The hunger for love is much more difficult to remove than
the hunger for bread.
~Mother Teresa

Mankind is important to God. We were born guilty due
to sin, but he redeemed us through his son. When we
accept Jesus, we are no longer guilty! This is some good
news for all of us. Tell me CHURCH why are we making
people feel guilty? Our job is to teach the Word of God and
it is the Holy Ghost's job to convict! God even said that he
did not send his Son into the world to judge the world but
through Him the world will be saved. Jesus is part of the
trinity which is the Father, Son and the Holy Ghost. The
Holy Ghost is the only one that can convict, Jesus knew what
his part was which was to walk on earth as a human soul and
then to die for our sins. If he was qualified to die for our
sins, (remember Jesus did not deserve to die because he
never did any wrong we did the wrong and we were the ones
who killed him as well) Jesus was qualified to convict. - No
condemnation When Jesus assented to heaven that is when
he became the Judge. (Remember this: Jesus was qualified to
convict but his Father did not send him here for that).
Therefore He did not judge! Neither should we!

He personally carried our sins in His body on the cross
(willingly offering Himself on it, as on an altar of sacrifice),
so that we might die to sin (becoming immune from the
penalty and power of sin) and live for righteousness ; for by
His wounds you (who believe) have been healed.
1 Peter 2:24 (AMP)

God knew we were sick and this is why His Son came was to heal the sick, raise the dead, heal the broken hearted and set the captive free. Jesus took everything on the cross with Him.

Unfortunately, the church has locked the doors on sinners this is contrary to God's plan. Yet, we are embarrassed if certain people come into our church such as homosexual, prostitute, cheater, drug addicts, drug dealers, alcoholic, teen parent, and etc. We do not represent God when we condemn the very ones his son died to save. Like us, they need to hear the TRUTH. We, the Church, is the hospital and have a duty to minister and teach the Word so God can operate.

It's easy to say—"Jesus loves sinners." Do we believe it? Not just for someone else, but do we believe it FOR OURSELVES? Jesus doesn't just love sinners in some generic, abstract way. It's not just about all those OTHER people. Jesus loves you. Jesus loves me. He loves the porn the racist, the murderer, the gossip, the homosexual, and the liar just to name a few because we know that there are many more. He loves all of us, right now—broken, sinful, lost, found. Period. **This does not mean He loves their sin**! He hates SIN no matter what it is, but HE loves SINNERS. There is a difference.

Have you ever wondered if the way the world is going today that God himself did this to bring back LOVE? We say we serve an all-powerful and knowing God. If this is so, then that means God already knew we would be in this place today. God is bringing his LOVE back to the church. Yes, we have lost it! Church, it is time to welcome the LOVE of

Christ back to the house of God. With the return of love, we will gain sinners!

Love is what draws and people feel love right away. They know when it is fake or real. This is similar to children when they are born and long for their mother's love. If Jesus had to teach the sinners the right way, what about us? It is just like a child, if you do not teach them between right and wrong they will never know. We are like little children. If you notice Jesus referred to us as little children all the time. Sinners desire love also!

What is our job as the Church? It's our job to teach the word of God and serve as the walking bible so others see Jesus within us. Jesus told his disciples to follow him. What if we tell someone to follow us? Are we setting a great example as God's disciple or are we living a double life? We, the church, are sometimes confused! Jesus said live HOLY for I am HOLY. Yes, we are not perfect, but we serve a perfect God and only through him are we made perfect. Our flesh is subject to do anything without God in our lives. If we renew our minds daily and stay before the Lord, do we not know that God will keep us. However, some of us don't want to be kept because we like living double lives. But saints; now it is up to us to become a great disciple for God! He is waiting for us to take our rightful place in the body of Christ.

John 4:19 "Come, follow me," Jesus said, "and I will send you out to fish for people.

His Love Is Inexhaustible

Consider this—Noah was a drunk, Moses was a murderer, King David was an adulterer and murderer, the Apostle Paul hunted and killed Christians, yet God loved them all and worked through them for His glory and their good. Jesus specifically loved and forgave the soldiers who tortured Him. They spit on Him; He loved them. They whipped Him; He loved them. They beat Him; He loved them. Eventually they killed Him, but He still loved them. Nothing they did to Him could stop His love for them.

> *[7-10] My beloved friends, let us continue to love each other since love comes from God. Everyone who loves is born of God and experiences a relationship with God. The person who refuses to love doesn't know the first thing about God, because God is love—so you can't know him if you don't love. This is how God showed his love for us: God sent his only Son into the world so we might live through him. This is the kind of love we are talking about—not that we once upon a time loved God, but that he loved us and sent his Son as a sacrifice to clear away our sins and the damage they've done to our relationship with God.*
> *1 John 4:7-10 (MSG)*

LOVE IS IMPORTANT TO GOD!

It says, "if you don't love, you don't know God" I am going to let that soak in for a moment. If you don't love, you don't know God…..ask yourself is there anyone you do not love? If so, you don't know God! Think about that!

This LOVE is so important to God that he says, without LOVE you have nothing. Meaning, you can go around preaching the gospel and speaking into others life, healing the sick, raising the died, helping the world but without

LOVE, none of these things mean anything to God! Now, this right here should awaken you today.

Love isn't just Jesus' behavior, it's His being. He loves because He is love and chooses to love us. He simply asks us to receive it.

The Power Of Love: Rahab's Case

God is powerful enough to make a difference in a sinner's life. If we read the Bible, we find that God purposed a prostitute named Rahab for his plan. Joshua sent two spies to scout out the city of Jericho for they were ready to take over the land by force. Rahab operated an inn built on the Jericho city wall where she hid the spies on her roof top. The fact is that Rahab sacrificed her life for her family and for Israel. Rahab showed love and courage because she was willing to lay down her life for her family and for the children of Israel. Remember Rahab lived in a city where they served idol gods. But Rahab told the spies that she had heard about their God! God knew the love Rahab had for her family. It's possible that everyone in her family didn't agree with her lifestyle and treat her with respect and love. Yet, she didn't think about that when she asked the spies to save her and her family. The love Rahab displayed was the love of Christ. Her love covered and was not selfish, envious, boastful, self-seeking, delighting in evil or prideful. The love Rahab displayed was patient, kind, protected, trusted and had hope not only for her but for her family. This type of love saved Rahab and her family!

No one expected God to give Rahab a place in his story.

My mother once inquired, "Why is it that the spies did not run to the CHURCH? Think about this and make your own notes of why the spies did not seek the church and then ask the Holy Ghost to reveal the real reason. I know some of you may say, there was no church Israel was the only one that served the true and living God and they were checking out the land. Rahab lived in a city where they served idol gods.

The expectation for the church is to serve as a place of safety, a place of trust, a place of peace, a place of happiness and healing. But yet in this story it was not the church that was used by God it was a prostitute. This is why we have to be careful and know that God will use whomever He likes and they just might not be from the church. When we as a Church think about others versus ourselves, then God can use us for special assignments.

God is challenging us to possess and deliver this Agape Love to others.

Take a moment to pray:

Father God, I thank you for loving me so much that you would send your only Son to die on the cross. Now Father I ask that you first forgive me if I have not displayed your love as I should have. I ask you now to give me unconditional love to display to this world so that they will see you within me and know that you love them no matter who they are or what they have done. Help me to love them back to health.

~

Notes

_____

_____

_____

_____

_____

_____

_____

_____

_____

_____

_____

_____

_____

_____

_____

_____

~CHAPTER 2~

THE WAY I SAW IT

Jesus' ministry was not limited to just the spiritual. He healed the sick, physical healing; he ministered to the brokenhearted, emotional healing; and he taught and preached, spiritual healing.

And Jesus went about all the cities and villages, teaching in their synagogues and preaching the gospel of the kingdom, and healing every sickness and every disease among the people.
Matthew 9:35

God spoke to me and said that the Church is like a hospital. Let's take a look at how a hospital operates and how this coincides with God loving us back to health. (I would like to just touch on a little information God shared with me to the church).

In Admissions, patients provide personal information and sign consent forms before going to a room or seeing a doctor. If the individual is critically ill, then, this information is usually obtained from a family member.

In addition to providing demographic and insurance information, patients receive a form explaining the HIPPA Law. What is the HIPPA Law? I am glad you asked. HIPPA stands for the Health Insurance Portability and Accountability Act and is a US law designed to provide privacy standards to protect patients' medical records and other health information provided to health plans, and other health care providers. In the explanation of HIPPA, two terms stand out for their importance. They are privacy and protection. Privacy refers to the state or condition of being free from being observed or disturbed by other people. With protection, it means to keep safe from harm or injury.

Now let's deal with the church not protecting the privacy of the people that are led by God to join their congregation. The members mistrust the leaders or anyone in the congregation because there has been hurt and backbiting in the so-called house of God! God's church should function as a place of security and safety. A place where anyone can come, confide in the leadership, and receive love rather than judgment from the leadership and the congregation. This is where the LOVE factor of Christ comes into play!!!! Love COVERS and PROTECTS …That's what the Love of God does!

As people enter the doors of the church, it is important for us to have a **spirit of protection for all people that are** connected in or out of church. This spirit creates a place where people feel safe and will not be judge for what they have done and who they are at any given time. Do we agree with their sins? NO, but it's our job to LOVE them back to Health and back to Righteousness! Who are we to say that God will not use a sinner. If God used us, then yes He can use anyone.

Moreover, we must keep information about our converts confidential since revealing such information about them could destroy the relationship established between the soul-winner and the convert. By so doing, we help new believers remain in the body of Christ. A reward awaits us if we would do.

As a patient, there are times when needles are inject to provide fluid or shots are administered. The needle prick is uncomfortable and sometimes painful. The same can occur in the church. When we are hurt by the church, our reaction may result in leaving the church. Before following through on the plan, know that God has faced hurt from us, but he never turned his back on us. Have you ever thought about how you hurt God by rejecting him? Yet, He loved you back to health and you go right back and do the very thing that you promised Him you would not do! I'll be honest. At one point, that was me. Yes, He opened His arms again and again for me and continued to LOVE me back to Health and back into my rightful place in Him. Just thinking about this brings me to tears because it is so many times I have turned my back on God, but He did not give up on me.

Listen, Church stop giving up on people that walk in and say they want to change, but we know their lifestyle and background! God is a forgiving God and unless they hear the TRUTH they will not come out of what they are in! It is our job to teach the TRUTH and not our opinions.

Unfortunately, the church is good about promoting their opinions and presenting it as truth. God's Word stands alone and doesn't need any assistance. The word of God says that God's ways are not our ways and his thoughts are not our thoughts.(Isaiah 55:8) Therefore, removing personal thoughts to welcome all those who come into the house of God enables God to deliver sinners and love them back to health.

It's common for people to go into an environment that they feel accepted versus one environment that makes them feel unwanted. If a brother or sister falls it is our duty to lift their arms. We become the encourager and love them back to their rightful place. What is their rightful place? Back into the Kingdom of God!

For I know the plans I have for you," declares the Lord, "plans to prosper you and not to harm you, plans to give you hope and a future.

Jeremiah 29:11 (NIV)

My question to you: Who was protecting her? Who is protecting the sinners of this world who wants to change their life?

In John 8:1-15, the scribes and Pharisees brought a woman, who had been caught in adultery, to Jesus. Now where was the man, who committed the adulterous act with her? Obviously, she was not alone. Nevertheless, they told Jesus about the law and asked Jesus for a verdict in this case. Isn't that just like the religious nuts! This is what we do to others sometimes. We bring people before the Lord and tell God all about their faults and failure, but totally forget about the errors we've made. The individuals joined the church and desired to know God. They connected with others in the church, who defamed them rather than serving as a support. This created a stressful situation resulting in the new member exiting the church and potentially crippling the relationship with God.

Rather than judging, we should ask God to have mercy on all of us. What if God exposed everything about us? Look at what Jesus said, "Let him who is without sin among you be the first to throw a stone at her." Once everyone dropped their stone and left individually, Jesus asked the woman, "Where are your accusers? Has no man condemned you? To her surprise, there was no one to accuse her. Along with the religious leaders, Jesus didn't accuse her either. Jesus was qualified to judge but he did not! He instead gave her direction for the rest of her life.

Wake up saints!!! It is time to become like Jesus and time to obtain and exhibit a spirit of protection. Love covers and protects.

We go to the hospital when you are sick, hurting and/or dying a desire to get healed so we can return back to our normal life. The hospital is not about to share our medical and/or personal information with anyone that does not have permission. If a person's name is not on the paperwork, the hospital doesn't care if it is your mother, father, husband and/or children. They will not share information about them with you. The Church should operate the same way. People are spiritually dying, hurting, and sick; they're in need of healing. We should never expose any private information to anyone about another person. Again I say, love protects and love covers. If this is the case, we should never have a problem protecting each other. It seems to me that the people in the church can't wait to expose each other but yet we say we have the love of Jesus. What if the hospital exposed our business to the world or others, we would be ready to sue the hospital. What if you could sue the church? It would be a lot of suing going on today! This is why people hold things in and are stressed right in the church! The church is a place of rest and peace, but we are stressed! Why? Because we are afraid to talk to anyone because we feel that our conversation will not be protected. Church we have to change this immediately and the only way we can change this if we take on the LOVE of Jesus because His love covers and protects.

Emergency Room

Emergency Room (ER) is a medical treatment facility specializing in emergency medicine, the acute care of patients who present without prior appointment; either by their own means or by that of an ambulance. The emergency department is usually found in a hospital or other primary care center. Due to the unplanned nature of patient attendance, the department must provide initial treatment for a broad spectrum of illnesses and injuries. Some may be life-threatening and require immediate attention. In some cases, emergency departments have become important entry points for those without other means of access to medical care.

The emergency departments of most hospitals operate 24 hours a day, although staffing levels may be varied in an attempt to reflect patient volume.

Some people suddenly get sick and need to see what is going on right away because they are uncertain about the source of their sickness or pain. If the doctor feels that the patients issue is worse and they need to have longer care, they prepare a room for the patient. If it is a major issue that will cost them their life and they need to monitor them, they will put the patient in the Intensive Care Unit (ICU) with the goal of restoring help.

Take A Moment To Pray:

Father God, thank you for covering and protecting me.
Forgive me for not doing the same for others as I should.
Please teach me how to protect and cover my brothers and
sisters in Christ. I thank you for your guidance to the right
path for my life and that of others.

Notes

~CHAPTER 3~

HELPING TO RESTORE LIFE

God loves you just the way you are, but He refuses to leave you that way. He wants you to be just like Jesus. – Max Lucado

As for the spiritual side, some people require immediate treatment to find the issue and God gives them a message for their healing. When individuals present with life threatening issues, the church assesses them in the ICU of the ministry and monitor them for safety. Others may need surgery; meaning, they receive daily doses of the Word of God. They eat the Word multiple times daily to restore them to health and equip them to stand on their own.

In the church, everyone is a servant and should be prepared to work 24/7 in order to remain equipped to deal with any sort of emergencies at any time. Until the issue is diagnosed, the problem cannot be treated. Most of the time we are all in a different place. Some of us need more care than others. It's the responsibility of the church to recognize and discern the needs of the people and assist them in moving forward.

This is why bible study is very important. The more we read the Word of God, the stronger we become. The more we love on everyone, the stronger we get.

The more truth we hear, the more it will cause us to change. If we don't like the medicine or prescribed course of treatment, we can leave the hospital without a proper discharge. Such measures can cause a reoccurrence of the original problem or make matters worse. It's always best to finish the treatment in order to experience complete healing. As it is in the natural, it is in the spiritual and bible study allows this to happen.

> [54-56] *"And when his disciples James and John saw this, they said, Lord, wilt thou that we command fire to come down from heaven, and consume them, even as Elias did? But He turned, and rebuked them, and said, Ye know not what manner of spirit ye are of. For the Son of man is not come to destroy men's lives, but to save them. And they went to another village."*
> *Luke 9:54-56*

In Luke 9:54-56, we find James and John eager to destroy the wicked with the wrath of God, but Jesus rebuked them instead, And likewise those profess they're Christians, but insist that God hates sinners... In case we aren't aware, only the spirit of Satan would reject the very one Jesus came to save. Jesus entered this world to save sinners; not to hate or destroy men's lives.

There are only two Scriptures in the New Testament where Jesus said "I hate" and they are Revelation 2:6 and 2:15.

> *"But this thou hast, that thou hatest the deeds of the Nicolaitans, which I also hate."*
> *Revelation 2:6*

> *"So hast thou also them that hold the doctrine of the Nicolaitans, which thing I hate."*
> *Revelation 2:15*

Jesus said that He hated the "deeds" of the Nicolaitans, and their "doctrine." Please notice that Jesus DIDN'T say He hated the Nicolaitans (a false cult). Jesus loves all sinners, not because they are sinners, but because they are people with souls.

"For God so loved the world, that he gave his only begotten Son, that whosoever believeth in him should not perish, but have everlasting life."
John 3:16

The "world" includes EVERYBODY, even a dirty, rotten, vile sinner like us. We stand against all types of wickedness, heresies, and sins yet proclaim the Biblical truth that God loves ALL people. No matter what they have done. That's not to say that God approves of their wickedness. It means that God unconditionally loves people. In the natural, I may not like all the choices my children make, but I will always love them. God does the same on a higher level.

Even after being nailed to a cross, Jesus expressed forgiveness to the Roman soldiers who had stripped him naked, beat Him beyond recognition, placed a sharp crown of thorns upon His head, mocked and spit on Him and then nailed Him to a cross to bleed and die (Luke 23:34). Don't you tell me that God doesn't love sinners! There is no depth of sin known to man, which can prevent the arm of God from saving the sinner who seeks forgiveness,

"Behold, the LORD's hand is not shortened, that it cannot save; neither his ear heavy, that it cannot hear: But your iniquities have separated between you and your God..."
Isaiah 59:1

If Jesus saved a murderer like Saul, who later became the Apostle Paul, then he will save anybody! If Jesus saved a drunkard like Noah, then He will save anybody. If Jesus saved an adulterer like David, then He will save anybody. This list goes on and on.

God receives any repentant sinner that comes to Jesus Christ for salvation (John 6:37). Repentance doesn't mean to turn from sin, but rather to change one's mind from what you want to do to what God says that you must do. God's way is through faith alone in Christ's death on the cross for our sins, His burial, and resurrection. This is the Gospel or good news. We are saved by believing the Gospel, by receiving Christ's sacrifice on the cross as full payment for our sins. If we go through difficulties and we will, but it is better to have trails and tribulations with God than without Him. When we deal with issues and have God on our side, this is where we will find peace that passes all understanding. But if we don't have God in our lives, stress, worry, crazy, and ungodly thoughts will take place. Believe on the Lord Jesus Christ and the work is done.

"Then said they unto him, What shall we do, that we might work the works of God? Jesus answered and said unto them, This is the work of God, that ye believe on him whom he hath sent."
John 6:28-29

What a tragedy that some people in the world will one day burn in the Lake of Fire, forfeiting the free gift of eternal life, which is already paid in full by Jesus' precious blood (1Peter 1:18,19).

Believe on Jesus as your Savior and you are saved!

He Cares for Us All

Jesus talked about His ministry in two ways. In Luke 4:18, He says, "The Spirit of the Lord is upon Me because He has anointed Me." He also talked about preaching the good news to the poor and the captive. Jesus came to serve. In fact, this type of ministry was a sign that He was the Messiah. He fulfilled prophecy as He showed kindness to those who were hurting. Throughout scripture, we see the work of Christ among the widows, the blind, the broken—whoever had a need. Jesus served with compassion. He came to save.

In Luke 19:10, Jesus says, "He came to seek and save the lost." And the same Jesus, who came to serve and to save then says to us in John 20:21, "As the Father has sent Me, I also send you." It is not how much we know, but how much we love.

Jesus sends us out to join Him in His mission. We are to serve others in His name, and to share the good news of salvation so that people might trust in Jesus' work on the cross—His death in our place, for our sin.

Serving and saving were marks of Christ's life on earth. They serve as marks of His people as well. But to do that, we must engage the broken and hurting people around us. A church that exemplifies Christ is one where broken people are welcome—a place where perfect people aren't allowed, where people can embark on their journey without having everything figured out from the start.

Don't leave them yet!

It is a natural thing for Christians to want to be around other Christians. Something special happens in the fellowship of believers. We worship freely, study deeply, and communicate clearly. Hanging out with like-minded people is a wonderful thing. But how well are we engaging those who aren't as spiritually stable as we think we are? *A church without the broken is a broken church.* How do we engage the hurting? Are we insulating ourselves from the brokenness around us? Are we so concerned about how people view us that we'll never be accused of spending too much time with sinners?

It's interesting that a lot of Christians don't seem to like non-Christians. These are those who are labeled as "the lost," "the unchurched," or whatever other term we may want to use. These so-called Christians want to keep away from the messy people, but miss the obvious that we are messy as well.

After coming to Christ and growing in knowledge, we often end up distancing ourselves from some of our former friends. We find that we have less and less time for the hurting and struggling because we're so "spiritual". We find the one thing that meets the need in our lives, but use it to block others from finding what they need God meets our needs and we move on, oblivious to the fact that the world is falling apart all around us. That is not the way of Christ.

Jesus lived differently. One of the common criticisms Jesus faced was that He spent too much time with sinners. He associated with the unwelcomed and unappreciated of society. How many of us could be accused of spending too much time with the "riff raff?"

> *"One of the Pharisees asked him over for a meal. He went to the Pharisee's house and sat down at the dinner table. Just then a woman of the village, the town harlot, having learned that Jesus was a guest in the home of the Pharisee, came with a bottle of very expensive perfume and stood at his feet, weeping, raining tears on his feet. Letting down her hair, she dried his feet, kissed them, and anointed them with the perfume. When the Pharisee who had invited him saw this, he said to himself, "If this man was the prophet I thought he was, he would have known what kind of woman this is who is falling all over him."*
> *Luke 7:36-39 (MSG)*

In the passage, the Pharisee had an issue with Jesus allowing the harlot anointing Jesus feet. My question was why would a harlot come to the Pharisee's home uninvited unless she knew them very well. My God from heaven. I really asked this question because no one with her background simply shows up at your home unless you know them very well. Think about it! I wonder if she was rubbing anyone else's feet except Jesus, would they have had a problem with her? I am just saying...my owe side note.

> *Jesus said to him, "Simon, I have something to tell you." "Oh? Tell me."* [41-42] *"Two men were in debt to a banker. One owed five hundred silver pieces, the other fifty. Neither of them could pay up, and so the banker canceled both debts. Which of the two would be more grateful?"* [43-47] *Simon answered, "I suppose the one who was forgiven the most."*

"That's right," said Jesus. Then turning to the woman, but speaking to Simon, he said, "Do you see this woman? I came to your home; you provided no water for my feet, but she rained tears on my feet and dried them with her hair. You gave me no greeting, but from the time I arrived she hasn't quit kissing my feet. You provided nothing for freshening up, but she has soothed my feet with perfume. Impressive, isn't it? She was forgiven many, many sins, and so she is very, very grateful. If the forgiveness is minimal, the gratitude is minimal."
*[48] Then he spoke to her: **"I forgive your sins."***
[49] That set the dinner guests talking behind his back: "Who does he think he is, forgiving sins!"[50] He ignored them and said to the woman, "Your faith has saved you. Go in peace."
Luke 7:40-51 (MSG)

And when the scribes and Pharisees saw him eat with publicans and sinners, they said unto his disciples, How is it that he eateth and drinketh with publicans and sinners? When Jesus heard it, he saith unto them, They that are whole have no need of the physician, but they that are sick: I came not to call the righteous, but sinners to repentance.
Mark 2:16-17

Here we have Jesus saying He came for the sick. If we are not sick, we do not need a physician. We only go to the doctor if we are sick. If we're doing well we may only need a yearly checkup. The church is looking only for well people! Wrong focus! We need to go find the sick and lost. It is easy to minister to someone that already knows Christ, but what about someone that never heard of Christ. We don't even speak about our Jesus at work but we will allow everyone to talk about everything else while we are afraid to talk about the one who died for ALL of our sins. Church we have to refocus. Love is the key. Once we fit this in the door, we are going to be able to unlock a lot of hearts and bring them to Christ. What I love about Jesus, He always gave instructions of what He needed the sinner to do next for example: go and sin no more.

What is so amazing is the so called church will cross people off in a heartbeat if they are not doing what we feel that they should do and how they should do it. It is amazing if a leader, singer, evangelist, prophet, teacher and/or pastor fall, the church turns their back and say to the world, "that is a shame what they did. I knew they did not have anything"! Stop it!!! We act sinless, but the fact is that we haven't been exposed yet. The church should pray for them in their fall. But oh no we have so much to say and we have others talking about things for which they have no clue. Are we in agreement with the sin? No, we are not but should we turn our backs on them? No, when they fall, they need us to hold their arms up. Love and tell them that God is a forgiving and loving God. Do you not know that we wouldn't have ex-preachers, ex-evangelist, ex-prophets, ex-pastors and ex-apostle if we would love people back to health!

Take A Moment To Pray:

Father God, I pray that I become a conduit for your love to stream out to others with whom I come in contact with on a day to day basis. I don't have all the answers but I want to continue to have your love.   Create in me a clean heart and renew the right spirit within me. Make me a **love tool for you.** When others are in need of your love allow me to be the tool that they will need to move forward into their new destiny. Let your love bounce off of me into them. Amen

Notes

~CHAPTER 4~

AGAPE LOVE TOWARDS EACH OTHER

<u>"YOU CAN SEE GOD FROM ANYWHERE IF YOUR MIND IS SET
TO LOVE AND OBEY HIM" ~ A.W. TOZER</u>

D*ear Church,*

*I have just become a Christian. I have confessed that I
love the Lord with all my heart etc., and I have determined to
do all things that are related by that statement. I have
determined to follow His instructions, commands, examples,
etc.. I have determined to rid my life of sin.
Is that enough? Do I really need to associate with the other
members of the church too: Do I need to hang around with
them? I don't even know most of them, do I need to like them
too, and get involved with them?*

Sincerely,

The Brethren and Unsaved

The simple answer is YES!

[22]Seeing ye have purified your souls in obeying the truth
through the Spirit unto unfeigned love of the brethren, see
that ye love one another with a pure heart fervently: [23]Being
born again, not of corruptible seed, but of incorruptible, by
the word of God, which liveth and abideth for ever. [24]For all
flesh is as grass, and all the glory of man as the flower of
grass. The grass withereth, and the flower thereof falleth
away: [25]But the word of the Lord endureth for ever. And this
is the word which by the gospel is preached unto you.
1 Peter 1:22-25

Brotherly Love Is Evidence Of Our Re-Birth.

If we are saved, where is our love for the other members of the church? Even if we are angry at them? Even if we're hurt by them? YES, folks will know we are Christians by our love. The inner rebirth that has taken place will be evident and obvious. What is the physical, visible evidence of God's love? Sincere love.

Some translations = "from a pure heart". Literally; "Without-hypocrisy"! Not in words only. Not in good pleasant thoughts only. Not simply that "melted" look. It's a matter of deeds and behavior. Not simply in nice emotions, but with actions! Christianity is a true heart religion that is action oriented.

Faith is seen in deeds! James 2:18, "...I will show you my faith by what I do." What were we created for in the first place? Ephesians 2:10, "For we are God's workmanship, created in Christ Jesus to do good works, which God prepared in advance for us to do." Part of those "good works" is loving the brethren with actions! We are talking about a fervent love.

It is easy to have a half-hearted love or a "somewhat" love, but this is not the same. In this same verse, the NIV says "deeply". The word comes from a word meaning to stretch and strain like a clothesline holding up a heavy burden. Real exertion of power, energy. Picture a champion arm wrestler; eyes bulging in complete devotion & focus! Anything we do without a total involvement is not "fervent". We love watermelon, old cars, pork chops, but not fervently, not "deeply". Our lives do not get all involved, governed by those things. We should do things in Christian love! When we fervently and deeply love our children, it is seen in our deeds. We would give them our kidney if needed.

So What?

In God's intention, there is no such thing as a "renegade" Christian, which is defined as one with no interaction with other Christians. One simply off doing his or her own thing and not functioning as an active part of God's Church, helping it fulfill its God-given role. By God's intention, Christians are to sincerely, actively, fervently love one another.

I hope your love has become real and that it brings unity to the Lord's body and cross all barriers that Satan might set up. I hope it is a love to cross social classes, racial distinctions, educational divisions, tastes in music, hobbies, hurts, and anything else that might separate people. Demonstrate salvation by actively and genuinely loving all the other members of Christ's church.

In 1 Peter 1:22-25, by the power and authority of Almighty God, the Holy Apostle Peter here urges Christians to bring their love for other members of the church to a reality. A basic reasons for a sincere love of the brethren are evident.

The reason Peter brings out for our learning to genuinely love other members of the church is one that ought to touch our very heart strings. We need to learn what it means to love the brethren because such Love Is The Very Purpose Of Conversion! God has a purpose for providing a means of salvation.

Was it simply to get you to heaven? Or is there something more? Is there something He expects to accomplish through the "saved"? What does He want and expect from us as Christians?

This passage also mentions "obeying the truth", which is responding to the Gospel. Obedience to the Gospel results in Purification, which enables us to have love for the brethren. God intends for Christians to possess Christ-like and godly love and becomes a major focus when we're purified.

We are changed

That's the meaning of "conversion". It means "changed". Changed into what God planned for us. Not just a one-time thing, but constant continual growth into Christ-likeness. Sanctification!

Are we willing to change? Are we serious about it? Are we really "purified by the Truth, or are we still abiding in our old selves? Are you changed from old selfish self? From self with hidden agendas and motives?

1 John 4:8 tells us that "God is love." meaning this is how we are to change and imitate Him. Ephesians 5:1 reads, "Be imitators of God, therefore, as dearly loved children…" 1 Timothy 1:5 says, "The goal of this command is love, which comes from a pure heart and a good conscience and a sincere faith". Such transformation into love is the very purpose and goal of all that the Bible teaches.

- Draws us into one Body! Ephesians 4:4, "There is one body and one Spirit—just as you were called to one hope when you were called."

- Enables the parts of the body to function together. Romans 12:4-5, "Just as each of us has one body with many members, and these members do not all have the same function, so in Christ we who are many form one body, and each member belongs to all the others."

Teachers, encouragers, givers, hospitality, and others have a role in the body. We need each other to accomplish God's desires.

Love heals

- Love allows blunders. "Above all, love each other deeply, because love covers over a multitude of sins." (1 Peter 4:8)
- Overcomes prejudices. We have bloopers. Ask dumb questions. Lose words and patience. If I stumble, will you help me get up. Because of love.

Who has blundered and hurt us? Will we still love them? Sincerely? Fervently?

Love Encourages Forgiveness

Sincere love breaks down dividing walls, pride, anger, opinions, customs, and personality conflicts. It is also a divine quality, patterned after God's forgiveness. Love provides strength to the weak. 1 Thessalonians 5:14, "And we urge you, brothers, warn those who are idle, encourage the timid, help the weak, be patient with everyone." Who stands in need of this genuine brotherly love? We all do. Such love identifies the true Christian and the true church for other people.

> *"A new command I give you: Love one another. As I have loved you, so you must love one another. By this all men will know that you are my disciples, if you love one another."*
> *John 13:34-35*

Is it evident to the world that we love one another? Is it evident to other Christians? Is it evident to those you might normally despise or avoid? Can they see you have been purified? Is your sort of love simply the natural love such as exists between all humans? Remember thieves and liars have some type of love. Christian love is extraordinary. Invisible things are often demonstrated through visible responses in tangible ways. Have you ever seen an itch? But you know that if I am scratching, I have an itch. Eating reveals that I am hungry. Leg jouncing = I am nervous / anxious. Fidget = bored. Head nod = agreement. So is our conversion. Our outward behavior is the proof that our heart has been converted!

Take A Moment To Pray:

Father God, thank you for allowing me to have that Agape love towards everyone that I come in contact with. Let your love continue to reign in my life. I thank you for the compassion and the will to love. Amen.

Notes

~CHAPTER 5~

UNCONDITONAL LOVE

The way to love anything is to realize that it may be lost.
~G.K. Chesterton

*Turn, O backsliding children, saith the LORD; for I am
married unto you: and I will take you one of a city, and two
of a family, and I will bring you to Zion:*
Jeremiah 3:14

The individual Christian, the Christian leader or minister
and the church as a whole have a responsibility towards
the new believer and the backslider (Mt. 28:19; Jude 22, 23)
to ensure that they stand firm in the Lord. One major cause
of backsliding is a poor Christian foundation. It is therefore,
necessary that believers, church leaders, counselors,
evangelists and pastors, explain the nature of the Christian
journey (Eph. 6:10-18; Lk. 6:22, 14:26; Jn. 15:18). In
addition, they must ensure that discipleship classes are
available in order to provide them with a firm foundation in
Christ, and also bring them to a point where they can
'journey' on their own.

Maturity in the life of Christians is very important (Heb.
5:11-6:2). It is not enough to lead others to Christ.Our
additional responsibility is to make them disciples of Jesus
Christ by helping them grow in the Christian faith. Our
failure to do this has produced immature Christians, who are
polluting the church with false doctrine and destroying the
unity of the church. As a result, some people have left their

original churches to establish congregations of their own and are manipulating new believers by using various methods in the name of performing healing and miracles. In other instances, failure to bring new converts to the point of maturity has resulted in strife, envy and power struggle in the body of Christ.

We fail also in our duties as watchmen when it comes to the responsibility we have towards backsliders. Christians should avoid behaving like the older son in Luke 15:25-32 who "... became angry and refused to go in" (v. 28a, NIV) when the Prodigal Son had returned, and the household was throwing a feast for him. We desire for the world to change. Unfortunately, when backsliders return to the Christian faith, we become judgmental and suspicious. Jonah, for instance, became indignant when God decided to spare Nineveh in Jonah 4. Then God asked him, "But Nineveh has more than a hundred and twenty thousand people who cannot tell their right hand from their left, and many cattle as well. Should I not be concerned about that great city?" If God was so concerned about the cattle in Nineveh, how can we ignore the spiritual needs of repentant backsliders and sinners? The next time we feel like judging, remember the grace of God. Paul, the apostle, faced the challenge of being accepted as a repentant sinner. The disciples in Jerusalem did not believe that he had converted to Christianity (Acts 9:26). But when Barnabas introduced Paul to the disciples, they recognized him as a disciple of Jesus Christ.

Whenever a sinner returns home, we should rejoice and give him the necessary support and encouragement to help him grow in Christ Jesus. As Christians, we need to have a burden for the backslidden. We are called to "bear one another's burdens" (Gal. 6:2, NIV), "exhort one another

daily" (Heb. 10:25, NIV), as watchmen, to warn the wicked
(Ezekiel 33:7, 8). However, in our attempts to help the
backslidden "rise up", we have to make sure that we are
strong enough to avoid being influenced (Jude 22, 23). In
whatever circumstance or situation, our attitude towards the
backslidden should remain one of compassion, of love, and
of mercy (2 Thess. 3:6, 15).

Jesus still loves you

Do you know…

1. In spite of your mistakes, Jesus loves you.

2. Despite continuous mistakes, Jesus still loves you.

Maybe you don't believe this. Maybe someone told you that
your sin is too much—that Jesus can't love you anymore.
Maybe you believe that God doesn't just hate your sin, but
He hates YOU, too. The truth is, you can't stop Jesus from
loving you. Nothing you can do can stop God, so you're
powerless against the love of God in Jesus.

The LORD wants you to know "Yes, I have loved you with
an everlasting love; Therefore with lovingkindness I have
drawn you" (Jeremiah 31:3 NKJV). That is the truth about
God's love for you. Believe it, receive it and claim it. Take a
moment and look at the phrase "lovingkindness I have drawn
you." This is a powerful and true statement. This is not
reserved for moments when we do things right, but it

includes the times when we don't. So many times, we disappoint God but guess what, He never stops loving us.

Regardless of how people treat you, Jesus still loves you. He never turns his back on us when we say no. He doesn't disown us. He doesn't close the door on us and say that we're not welcome. We're simply not strong enough to block God's love.

When Jesus was on Earth, He spent so much time eating with sinners that the religious leaders accused Him of being a sinner. He wasn't—Jesus lived a perfect, sinless life to take our place, pay for our sins, and give us eternal, abundant life. He didn't encourage or condone the sin of the sinners seated around His dinner table. He wasn't ok with their sins, but He loved them and he knew they needed His help. He loved them, taught, encouraged, and built relationships with them. He did the same thing for them then that He does for us now.

When Jesus chose His disciples. he chose ALL SINNERS! WOW!!!! He never told them to lay down their sins. He told them to follow HIM. Jesus knew after teaching them the RIGHT WAY, they would have the opportunity to do what is right.

The Prodigal Son is a great story located in Luke 15:11-32. The Father represents our Father in heaven. Displaying the love, he has for you by forgiving and welcoming you back with open arms. The younger son symbolizes the lost and the elder brother represents the self-righteous. The son asked his father for all his stuff that is due to him (what you are going to give me now and when you are dead) now. The father gave him his portion and the son left. That is how some of us act with God. You ask God for everything and once he gives it to you, you leave and do your own thing.

The thing that I love about the Prodigal son story is that the Father loved his son so much that he waited for his son's return. God is waiting for your return. Why because He loves us so much! I am sure the people in town talked about the father and said how crazy he was for giving his son the biggest party ever! This is what Jesus does when you return to him.

 If God is all knowing then he knew the ride we're going to take. Because God is a gentleman, he will not kick our door down! Ruth and Orpah are great examples. These were two women, who married two brothers. Naomi was a believer and Ruth and Oprah was around her, but when Naomi's husband and two sons died the decision came for Ruth and Oprah to return to their homeland. Now both ladies were with the family the same amount of time but only ONE got it!!! Wow! This will preach because sometimes we feel as if everyone should receive at the same time but sometimes it does not happen that way.

Orpah decided to go back to her homeland and sometimes people will come and hear the same word but still decide to continue with the world. However, her decision didn't stop Naomi or God from loving her.

Ruth saw beyond herself and Naomi's situation.   She decided that not only does her mother-in-law love her but said "where she go I will go, where she stay I will stay her God is my God!" God's love is so strong until He will make sure your steps are ordered by Him. God ensured that Ruth would fulfill the assignment he had for her. When God has an assignment for you no devil in hell can stop it.

Naomi two sons married ladies that they should not have ever married BUT God! God wanted to use Ruth so He had to make sure she married in the right family and had the right mother in law! Ruth fulfilled her purpose. I am sure people talked about Naomi and her family of how her boys married those Moabite girls! This is why God is in control because we don't know the plans He has for us, but He knows. I am so glad He has a plan for our lives.

What do you do when others make it hard to love them? Is there such a thing as making it hard to love them? What if Jesus said that you are making it too hard for Him to love you? You would be in trouble.

The Church is not a perfect place for it is striving to exemplify Christ. There are times when the members of the Church are less than stellar; however, place your focus on God and allow him to minister to you in all situations. Just like He did for me, He will show you how to love those who have harmed you. Therefore, you have a responsibility to ensure that you maintain your confession of faith despite the situation.

This season in my life God has challenged my Love with others. Yes, a lot of things hurt me during this time but guess what I had to love any way. I know you are saying, "how do you love someone that is always plotting to kill you"? Well, I am here to tell you if your love is real, God will not allow them to kill you or allow you to fall in the hole that they plotted for you. What God will do is EXPOSE the plot. In the book of Esther, Haman plotted to kill the King but Esther received a message about that very plot! Mordecai was a man that stayed before God, stayed in God's face fasting and praying. If you are doing this, you can rest assure that God is going to reign on your behalf! This is good news for you. Praise Him right there! Glory!

Many times, you feel that God doesn't see or hear what the enemy is doing, but I came to remind you that God knows ALL and SEES ALL. Even when Mordecai informed Esther of the two servants that plotted to kill the King. God did not allow the King to reward Mordecai until the appointed time that it was needed to show the enemy that He (God) is in control of ALL things. So in the meantime you did not hear Mordecai bad mouth Haman or bow to Haman because his allegiance was to God. Mordecai prayed and fasted before God.

I can imagine Mordecai's love for God was so strong until he did not have time to go after the enemy. That is how strong your love should be with God. When you love Him, then He will pour His love into you so you can love others, even your enemy.

Let's Take A Moment To Pray:

Father God, I pray that you give me the compassion for others just as you have given to me. I can not do this on my own so I pray that you will search my heart and if you find anything that is not willing to love like you, please remove. Just as your love brought us all back to health allow someone else to experience that love so that they may come back into their rightful place in you. Let them feel the love as they walk into your presence. Amen

Notes

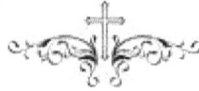

What has been amazing to me is that the world will have your back when the so called saints will drag others name down and we are the one that should be holding each other up. This is one of the reasons that I hear sinners say they hate coming to church. They see the church fighting against each other.

After reading this book, you should say to yourself, "Self, if I don't have anything good to say, then I won't say anything especially about the people of God". If you can't help them, leave them alone. Have you ever thought that maybe people don't know a better way; they are only doing it the way they have been taught. We can assist by teaching them a different and right way.

The church is so mean is what I always hear from sinners! Why is this? Because we are not nice, we are always talking about people or things that we should not talk about and we only want to see our church succeed when it should be where we want the Kingdom of God to succeed. If one church hurt we all should hurt. If one church is successful, we all should feel successful. But we have to begin to operate like the Kingdom of Heaven, which he designed to be on earth for us. Thy Kingdom come thy will be done on earth as it is in heaven.

God's original plan was for all of us to be with Him in heaven. We have to show and display the Love of God on a day to day basis by loving people back to health.

When we "The Church" begin to show each other love and display the Agape Love we will win souls. He who winneth souls are wise (Proverbs 11:30). Remember, we are nothing without Love. Let it be who you are. We should be remembered by our love, not our name, not our job, not our gift or talent but by our LOVE!

Notes

~7 DAY AGAPE LOVE CHALLENGE~

Please take time during your day for the next (7) seven days to complete the following questions. They are designed to help you focus and reflect on the fundamental issues you need to consider as you begin your journey of love.

Day #1

Love is Patient

How did you display patient on today?

_____

_____

_____

_____

_____

Was it or how was it difficult for you?

_____

_____

_____

_____

_____

Day #2

Love is Kind

How did you display kindness on today?

_____

_____

_____

_____

Was it or how was it difficult for you?

_____

_____

_____

_____

Day #3

Love is not jealous or envious

How did you display not being jealous or envious on today?

_____

_____

_____

_____

Was it or how was it difficult for you?

_____

_____

_____

_____

_____

Day #4

Love does not brag and is not proud or arrogant.

How did you display not bragging and having proud on today.

_____

_____

_____

Was it or how was it difficult for you?

_____

_____

_____

_____

_____

Day #5

Love is not rude.

How did you display not being rude to anyone on today?

_____

_____

_____

_____

_____

Was it or how was it difficult for you?

_____

_____

_____

_____

_____

Day #6

Love covers and protects.

Did your love cover and protected anyone on today.?

_____

_____

_____

_____

_____

Was it or how was it difficult for you?

_____

_____

_____

_____

_____

Day #7

Love puts up with anything, trusts God always, always looks for the best, never looks back but keeps going to the end.

How did you handle putting up with everything, trusting God, looking for the best in every situation without looking back and going to the end?

_____

_____

_____

_____

Was it or how was it difficult for you?

_____

_____

_____

_____

<u>LOVE</u>

L –What is it that you need to ***<u>Let Go</u>*** to start your agape love journey

O – What is it that you need to ***<u>Overcome</u>*** so that you can begin to have that Agape love

V – Make a ***<u>Vow to love</u>***

E – How can you ***<u>Express</u>*** the love of Christ daily

_____

_____

_____

_____

_____

_____

_____

_____

_____

_____

_____

_____

~AFTERWORD~

There is no greater power than the power of LOVE. Love is what lifts us and brings us back to health. As I continue to say, His Son came not to judge but to LOVE.

I challenge you to go to your churches, schools, homes, and work places, and begin to use the love that God has bestowed upon you. Go ahead because God believes in you! I challenge you to make a difference in someone's life every single day. Make up your mind to Love daily, and remember to imitate Christ.

Love is your destiny! Love will cover! Love will heal! Love will protect! Love does not envy! Love with joy! Love with compassion! Love, love, love! Ask yourself, "Who am I going to Love Back to Health today?" No matter how they treat you, Love them! Don't forget that God loved us first!

We have no right to continue to kill each other with our tongue, our thoughts and/or looks. If we are going to displace God and show others His love, we must change by reflecting the love of Christ. He is a God who gives so much love and continues to heal our hearts, not just the world but each and every one of us.

My deep and sincere desire is that by sharing what God has given me will empower you to display the Agape Love.

REMEMBER TO LOVE OTHERS BACK TO HEALTH!

Evangelist Mary Rieves

A conversation on love is incomplete without a biblical discussion of God's love. This is the love that leads to a path for eternal life. Praise God!

Below are several scriptures which showcase love and how it affects our lives.

For God so loved the world, that he gave his only Son, that whoever believes in him should not perish but have eternal life.
John 3:16

But God shows his love for us in that while we were still sinners, Christ died for us.
Romans 5:8

No, in all these things we are more than conquerors through him who loved us. For I am sure that neither death nor life, nor angels nor rulers, nor things present nor things to come, nor powers, nor height nor depth, nor anything else in all creation, will be able to separate us from the love of God in Christ Jesus our Lord.
Romans 8:37-39

I have been crucified with Christ. It is no longer I who live, but Christ who lives in me. And the life I now live in the flesh I live by faith in the Son of God, who loved me and gave himself for me.
Galatians 2:20

See what kind of love the Father has given to us, that we should be called children of God; and so we are. The reason why the world does not know us is that it did not know him.
1 John 3:1

Owe no one anything, except to love each other, for the one who loves another has fulfilled the law.
Romans 13:8

For you were called to freedom, brothers. Only do not use your freedom as an opportunity for the flesh, but through love serve one another.
Galatians 5:13

With all humility and gentleness, with patience, bearing with one another in love.
Ephesians 4:2
Having purified your souls by your obedience to the truth for a sincere brotherly love, love one another earnestly from a pure heart,
1 Peter 1:22

Beloved, let us love one another, for love is from God, and whoever loves has been born of God and knows God.
1 John 4:7

"You have heard that it was said, 'You shall love your neighbor and hate your enemy.' But I say to you, Love your enemies and pray for those who persecute you, so that you may be sons of your Father who is in heaven. For he makes his sun rise on the evil and on the good, and sends rain on the just and on the unjust. For if you love those who love you, what reward do you have? Do not even the tax collectors do the same? And if you greet only your brothers,

*what more are you doing than others? Do not even the
Gentiles do the same? You therefore must be perfect, as your
heavenly Father is perfect.*
Matthew 5:43-48

*"No one can serve two masters, for either he will hate the
one and love the other, or he will be devoted to the one and
despise the other. You cannot serve God and money.
"Therefore I tell you, do not be anxious about your life, what
you will eat or what you will drink, nor about your body,
what you will put on. Is not life more than food, and the body
more than clothing?*
Matthew 6:24-25

*And one of the scribes came up and heard them disputing
with one another, and seeing that he answered them well,
asked him, "Which commandment is the most important of
all?" Jesus answered, "The most important is, 'Hear, O
Israel: The Lord our God, the Lord is one. And you shall
love the Lord your God with all your heart and with all your
soul and with all your mind and with all your strength.'*
Mark 12:28-30

*Whoever has my commandments and keeps them, he it is who
loves me. And he who loves me will be loved by my Father,
and I will love him and manifest myself to him." Judas (not
Iscariot) said to him, "Lord, how is it that you will manifest
yourself to us, and not to the world?" Jesus answered him,
"If anyone loves me, he will keep my word, and my Father
will love him, and we will come to him and make our home
with him. Whoever does not love me does not keep my words.
And the word that you hear is not mine but the Fathers who
sent me.*
John 14:21-24

As the Father has loved me, so have I loved you. Abide in my love. If you keep my commandments, you will abide in my love, just as I have kept my Father's commandments and abide in his love. These things I have spoken to you, that my joy may be in you, and that your joy may be full. "This is my commandment, that you love one another as I have loved you. Greater love has no one than this, that someone lay down his life for his friends. You are my friends if you do what I command you. No longer do I call you servants, for the servant does not know what his master is doing; but I have called you friends, for all that I have heard from my Father I have made known to you. You did not choose me, but I chose you and appointed you that you should go and bear fruit and that your fruit should abide, so that whatever you ask the Father in my name, he may give it to you. These things I command you, so that you will love one another.

John 15:9-17

~ABOUT THE AUTHOR~

Mary Rieves Pastor's with her husband Pastor Darrell Rieves at the Kingdom of God International Church located in Brandon, Florida. She is also the founder of Mary Rieves Ministries and the CEO of TAGIN, INC (Non-Profit Organization / www.tag-org.com).

Mary has been singing since she was a little girl. After almost losing her life, God spoke to Mary to record a gospel CD. Mary has released three CDs entitled "Hide Me," "I Trust You Lord," and "So Amazing".

Mary Rieves has been blessed to share her ministry on The Word Network, TBN Broadcasting, Streaming Faith Broadcasting, and Dr. Bobby Jones Gospel. She has shared the stage with Rickey Dillard, John P. Kee, Shirley Caesar, and Barbara Mitchell, to name a few. Mary has also traveled extensively sharing her music ministry at many gospel events, conferences, and services.

Mary is a worker for the Kingdom of God and she continues to humbly serve by staying obedient to the Word of God. She knows that she is anointed by God for such a time as this. Mary continues to move in His will by imitating Christ. She knows that she shall inherit the Kingdom of God! Mary's goal is to reach the lost, and let them know that Christ still loves and care for them. Although Mary has achieved much, the title that means the most to her is "Servant of God!"

Mary Rieves and her husband, Darrell Rieves, are the parents of three lovely children: Joshua, Naomi, and Rachel. Along with my three Glam Babies!

~

.

www.ingramcontent.com/pod-product-compliance
Lightning Source LLC
Chambersburg PA
CBHW060156070426
42447CB00033B/2181